Email us at

busyorganizerofficial@gmail.com

to get extra freebies!

Just title the email "**Running Log**"

And we will send some printable freebies

surprises your way!

2021

JANUARY

S	M	T	W	T	F	S
					1	2
3	4	5	6	7	8	9
10	11	12	13	14	15	16
17	18	19	20	21	22	23
24	25	26	27	28	29	30
31						

| JAN 1 | New Year's Day |
| JAN 18 | Martin Luther King Jr. Day |

FEBRUARY

S	M	T	W	T	F	S
	1	2	3	4	5	6
7	8	9	10	11	12	13
14	15	16	17	18	19	20
21	22	23	24	25	26	27
28						

FEB 1	First Day of Black History Month
FEB 14	Valentine's Day
FEB 15	Presidents' Day (Most regions)

MARCH

S	M	T	W	T	F	S
	1	2	3	4	5	6
7	8	9	10	11	12	13
14	15	16	17	18	19	20
21	22	23	24	25	26	27
28	29	30	31			

| MAR 1 | First Day of Women's History Month |
| MAR 17 | St. Patrick's Day |

APRIL

S	M	T	W	T	F	S
				1	2	3
4	5	6	7	8	9	10
11	12	13	14	15	16	17
18	19	20	21	22	23	24
25	26	27	28	29	30	

APR 4	Easter Sunday
APR 5	Easter Monday
APR 15	Tax Day

MAY

S	M	T	W	T	F	S
						1
2	3	4	5	6	7	8
9	10	11	12	13	14	15
16	17	18	19	20	21	22
23	24	25	26	27	28	29
30	31					

MAY 5	Cinco de Mayo
MAY 9	Mother's Day
MAY 31	Memorial Day

JUNE

S	M	T	W	T	F	S
		1	2	3	4	5
6	7	8	9	10	11	12
13	14	15	16	17	18	19
20	21	22	23	24	25	26
27	28	29	30			

| JUN 19 | Juneteenth |
| JUN 20 | Father's Day |

JULY

S	M	T	W	T	F	S
				1	2	3
4	5	6	7	8	9	10
11	12	13	14	15	16	17
18	19	20	21	22	23	24
25	26	27	28	29	30	31

| JUL 4 | Independence Day |
| JUL 5 | Independence Day observed |

AUGUST

S	M	T	W	T	F	S
1	2	3	4	5	6	7
8	9	10	11	12	13	14
15	16	17	18	19	20	21
22	23	24	25	26	27	28
29	30	31				

SEPTEMBER

S	M	T	W	T	F	S
			1	2	3	4
5	6	7	8	9	10	11
12	13	14	15	16	17	18
19	20	21	22	23	24	25
26	27	28	29	30		

| SEP 6 | Labor Day |

OCTOBER

S	M	T	W	T	F	S
					1	2
3	4	5	6	7	8	9
10	11	12	13	14	15	16
17	18	19	20	21	22	23
24	25	26	27	28	29	30
31						

| OCT 11 | Columbus Day (Most regions) |
| OCT 31 | Halloween |

NOVEMBER

S	M	T	W	T	F	S
	1	2	3	4	5	6
7	8	9	10	11	12	13
14	15	16	17	18	19	20
21	22	23	24	25	26	27
28	29	30				

NOV 2	Election Day
NOV 11	Veterans Day
NOV 25	Thanksgiving Day
NOV 26	Black Friday

DECEMBER

S	M	T	W	T	F	S
			1	2	3	4
5	6	7	8	9	10	11
12	13	14	15	16	17	18
19	20	21	22	23	24	25
26	27	28	29	30	31	

DEC 24	Christmas Day observed
DEC 24	Christmas Eve
DEC 25	Christmas Day
DEC 31	New Year's Day observed
DEC 31	New Year's Eve

2022

JANUARY

S	M	T	W	T	F	S
						1
2	3	4	5	6	7	8
9	10	11	12	13	14	15
16	17	18	19	20	21	22
23	24	25	26	27	28	29
30	31					

JAN 1	New Year's Day
JAN 17	Martin Luther King Jr. Day

FEBRUARY

S	M	T	W	T	F	S
		1	2	3	4	5
6	7	8	9	10	11	12
13	14	15	16	17	18	19
20	21	22	23	24	25	26
27	28					

FEB 1	First Day of Black History Month
FEB 14	Valentine's Day
FEB 21	Presidents' Day (Most regions)

MARCH

S	M	T	W	T	F	S
		1	2	3	4	5
6	7	8	9	10	11	12
13	14	15	16	17	18	19
20	21	22	23	24	25	26
27	28	29	30	31		

MAR 1	First Day of Women's History Month
MAR 17	St. Patrick's Day

APRIL

S	M	T	W	T	F	S
					1	2
3	4	5	6	7	8	9
10	11	12	13	14	15	16
17	18	19	20	21	22	23
24	25	26	27	28	29	30

APR 17	Easter Sunday
APR 18	Easter Monday
APR 18	Tax Day

MAY

S	M	T	W	T	F	S
1	2	3	4	5	6	7
8	9	10	11	12	13	14
15	16	17	18	19	20	21
22	23	24	25	26	27	28
29	30	31				

MAY 5	Cinco de Mayo
MAY 8	Mother's Day
MAY 30	Memorial Day

JUNE

S	M	T	W	T	F	S
			1	2	3	4
5	6	7	8	9	10	11
12	13	14	15	16	17	18
19	20	21	22	23	24	25
26	27	28	29	30		

JUN 19	Father's Day
JUN 19	Juneteenth

JULY

S	M	T	W	T	F	S
					1	2
3	4	5	6	7	8	9
10	11	12	13	14	15	16
17	18	19	20	21	22	23
24	25	26	27	28	29	30
31						

JUL 4	Independence Day

AUGUST

S	M	T	W	T	F	S
	1	2	3	4	5	6
7	8	9	10	11	12	13
14	15	16	17	18	19	20
21	22	23	24	25	26	27
28	29	30	31			

SEPTEMBER

S	M	T	W	T	F	S
				1	2	3
4	5	6	7	8	9	10
11	12	13	14	15	16	17
18	19	20	21	22	23	24
25	26	27	28	29	30	

SEP 5	Labor Day

OCTOBER

S	M	T	W	T	F	S
						1
2	3	4	5	6	7	8
9	10	11	12	13	14	15
16	17	18	19	20	21	22
23	24	25	26	27	28	29
30	31					

OCT 10	Columbus Day (Most regions)
OCT 31	Halloween

NOVEMBER

S	M	T	W	T	F	S
		1	2	3	4	5
6	7	8	9	10	11	12
13	14	15	16	17	18	19
20	21	22	23	24	25	26
27	28	29	30			

NOV 8	Election Day
NOV 11	Veterans' Day
NOV 24	Thanksgiving Day
NOV 25	Black Friday

DECEMBER

S	M	T	W	T	F	S
				1	2	3
4	5	6	7	8	9	10
11	12	13	14	15	16	17
18	19	20	21	22	23	24
25	26	27	28	29	30	31

DEC 24	Christmas Eve
DEC 25	Christmas Day
DEC 26	Christmas Day observed
DEC 31	New Year's Eve

GOALS

- [ ]
- [ ]
- [ ]
- [ ]
- [ ]
- [ ]
- [ ]
- [ ]
- [ ]
- [ ]
- [ ]
- [ ]
- [ ]
- [ ]
- [ ]
- [ ]
- [ ]
- [ ]
- [ ]
- [ ]
- [ ]
- [ ]
- [ ]
- [ ]
- [ ]
- [ ]
- [ ]
- [ ]
- [ ]

PERSONAL RECORD

DATE	RACE	DISTANCE	PR (PERSONAL RECORD)	PB (PERSONAL BEST)

BUCKET LIST RACES

DATE	RACE	LOCATION	DONE
			☐
			☐
			☐
			☐
			☐
			☐
			☐
			☐
			☐
			☐
			☐
			☐
			☐
			☐
			☐
			☐
			☐
			☐
			☐
			☐
			☐
			☐
			☐
			☐
			☐
			☐
			☐

BUCKET LIST RACES

DATE	RACE	LOCATION	DONE
			☐
			☐
			☐
			☐
			☐
			☐
			☐
			☐
			☐
			☐
			☐
			☐
			☐
			☐
			☐
			☐
			☐
			☐
			☐
			☐
			☐
			☐
			☐
			☐
			☐
			☐
			☐
			☐

MY RACES

DATE	RACE NAME	DISTANCE	TIME	PACE	PLACE NO.

MY RACES

DATE	RACE NAME	DISTANCE	TIME	PACE	PLACE NO.

SUMMARY

	WEEK	DISTANCE	NOTES
1	December 28, 2020 – January 3, 2021		
2	January 4, 2021 – January 10, 2021		
3	January 11, 2021 – January 17, 2021		
4	January 18, 2021 – January 24, 2021		
5	January 25, 2021 – January 31, 2021		
6	February 1, 2021 – February 7, 2021		
7	February 8, 2021 – February 14, 2021		
8	February 15, 2021 – February 21, 2021		
9	February 22, 2021 – February 28, 2021		
10	March 1, 2021 – March 7, 2021		
11	March 8, 2021 – March 14, 2021		
12	March 15, 2021 – March 21, 2021		
13	March 22, 2021 – March 28, 2021		
14	March 29, 2021 – April 4, 2021		
15	April 5, 2021 – April 11, 2021		
16	April 12, 2021 – April 18, 2021		
17	April 19, 2021 – April 25, 2021		
18	April 26, 2021 – May 2, 2021		
19	May 3, 2021 – May 9, 2021		
20	May 10, 2021 – May 16, 2021		
21	May 17, 2021 – May 23, 2021		
22	May 24, 2021 – May 30, 2021		
23	May 31, 2021 – June 6, 2021		
24	June 7, 2021 – June 13, 2021		
25	June 14, 2021 – June 20, 2021		
26	June 21, 2021 – June 27, 2021		

27	June 28, 2021 – July 4, 2021		
28	July 5, 2021 – July 11, 2021		
29	July 12, 2021 – July 18, 2021		
30	July 19, 2021 – July 25, 2021		
31	July 26, 2021 – August 1, 2021		
32	August 2, 2021 – August 8, 2021		
33	August 9, 2021 – August 15, 2021		
34	August 16, 2021 – August 22, 2021		
35	August 23, 2021 – August 29, 2021		
36	August 30, 2021 – September 5, 2021		
37	September 6, 2021 – September 12, 2021		
38	September 13, 2021 – September 19, 2021		
39	September 20, 2021 – September 26, 2021		
40	September 27, 2021 – October 3, 2021		
41	October 4, 2021 – October 10, 2021		
42	October 11, 2021 – October 17, 2021		
43	October 18, 2021 – October 24, 2021		
44	October 25, 2021 – October 31, 2021		
45	November 1, 2021 – November 7, 2021		
46	November 8, 2021 – November 14, 2021		
47	November 15, 2021 – November 21, 2021		
48	November 22, 2021 – November 28, 2021		
49	November 29, 2021 – December 5, 2021		
50	December 6, 2021 – December 12, 2021		
51	December 13, 2021 – December 19, 2021		
52	December 20, 2021 – December 26, 2021		
53	December 27, 2021 – January 2, 2022		
	TOTAL		

2021

JANUARY	FEBRUARY	MARCH	APRIL	MAY	JUNE
1 Fr	1 Mo	1 Mo	1 Th	1 Sa	1 Tu
2 Sa	2 Tu	2 Tu	2 Fr	2 Su	2 We
3 Su	3 We	3 We	3 Sa	3 Mo	3 Th
4 Mo	4 Th	4 Th	4 Su	4 Tu	4 Fr
5 Tu	5 Fr	5 Fr	5 Mo	5 We	5 Sa
6 We	6 Sa	6 Sa	6 Tu	6 Th	6 Su
7 Th	7 Su	7 Su	7 We	7 Fr	7 Mo
8 Fr	8 Mo	8 Mo	8 Th	8 Sa	8 Tu
9 Sa	9 Tu	9 Tu	9 Fr	9 Su	9 We
10 Su	10 We	10 We	10 Sa	10 Mo	10 Th
11 Mo	11 Th	11 Th	11 Su	11 Tu	11 Fr
12 Tu	12 Fr	12 Fr	12 Mo	12 We	12 Sa
13 We	13 Sa	13 Sa	13 Tu	13 Th	13 Su
14 Th	14 Su	14 Su	14 We	14 Fr	14 Mo
15 Fr	15 Mo	15 Mo	15 Th	15 Sa	15 Tu
16 Sa	16 Tu	16 Tu	16 Fr	16 Su	16 We
17 Su	17 We	17 We	17 Sa	17 Mo	17 Th
18 Mo	18 Th	18 Th	18 Su	18 Tu	18 Fr
19 Tu	19 Fr	19 Fr	19 Mo	19 We	19 Sa
20 We	20 Sa	20 Sa	20 Tu	20 Th	20 Su
21 Th	21 Su	21 Su	21 We	21 Fr	21 Mo
22 Fr	22 Mo	22 Mo	22 Th	22 Sa	22 Tu
23 Sa	23 Tu	23 Tu	23 Fr	23 Su	23 We
24 Su	24 We	24 We	24 Sa	24 Mo	24 Th
25 Mo	25 Th	25 Th	25 Su	25 Tu	25 Fr
26 Tu	26 Fr	26 Fr	26 Mo	26 We	26 Sa
27 We	27 Sa	27 Sa	27 Tu	27 Th	27 Su
28 Th	28 Su	28 Su	28 We	28 Fr	28 Mo
29 Fr		29 Mo	29 Th	29 Sa	29 Tu
30 Sa		30 Tu	30 Fr	30 Su	30 We
31 Su		31 We		31 Mo	

2021

JULY	AUGUST	SEPTEMBER	OCTOBER	NOVEMBER	DECEMBER
1 Th	1 Su	1 We	1 Fr	1 Mo	1 We
2 Fr	2 Mo	2 Th	2 Sa	2 Tu	2 Th
3 Sa	3 Tu	3 Fr	3 Su	3 We	3 Fr
4 Su	4 We	4 Sa	4 Mo	4 Th	4 Sa
5 Mo	5 Th	5 Su	5 Tu	5 Fr	5 Su
6 Tu	6 Fr	6 Mo	6 We	6 Sa	6 Mo
7 We	7 Sa	7 Tu	7 Th	7 Su	7 Tu
8 Th	8 Su	8 We	8 Fr	8 Mo	8 We
9 Fr	9 Mo	9 Th	9 Sa	9 Tu	9 Th
10 Sa	10 Tu	10 Fr	10 Su	10 We	10 Fr
11 Su	11 We	11 Sa	11 Mo	11 Th	11 Sa
12 Mo	12 Th	12 Su	12 Tu	12 Fr	12 Su
13 Tu	13 Fr	13 Mo	13 We	13 Sa	13 Mo
14 We	14 Sa	14 Tu	14 Th	14 Su	14 Tu
15 Th	15 Su	15 We	15 Fr	15 Mo	15 We
16 Fr	16 Mo	16 Th	16 Sa	16 Tu	16 Th
17 Sa	17 Tu	17 Fr	17 Su	17 We	17 Fr
18 Su	18 We	18 Sa	18 Mo	18 Th	18 Sa
19 Mo	19 Th	19 Su	19 Tu	19 Fr	19 Su
20 Tu	20 Fr	20 Mo	20 We	20 Sa	20 Mo
21 We	21 Sa	21 Tu	21 Th	21 Su	21 Tu
22 Th	22 Su	22 We	22 Fr	22 Mo	22 We
23 Fr	23 Mo	23 Th	23 Sa	23 Tu	23 Th
24 Sa	24 Tu	24 Fr	24 Su	24 We	24 Fr
25 Su	25 We	25 Sa	25 Mo	25 Th	25 Sa
26 Mo	26 Th	26 Su	26 Tu	26 Fr	26 Su
27 Tu	27 Fr	27 Mo	27 We	27 Sa	27 Mo
28 We	28 Sa	28 Tu	28 Th	28 Su	28 Tu
29 Th	29 Su	29 We	29 Fr	29 Mo	29 We
30 Fr	30 Mo	30 Th	30 Sa	30 Tu	30 Th
31 Sa	31 Tu		31 Su		31 Fr

JANUARY 2021

SUNDAY	MONDAY	TUESDAY	WEDNESDAY
3	4	5	6
10	11	12	13
17	18	19	20
24 31	25	26	27

THURSDAY	FRIDAY	SATURDAY	
	1	2	
7	8	9	
14	15	16	
21	22	23	
28	29	30	Jan 1 New Year's Day Jan 18 Martin Luther King Jr. Day

FEBRUARY 2021

SUNDAY	MONDAY	TUESDAY	WEDNESDAY
	1	2	3
7	8	9	10
14	15	16	17
21	22	23	24
28			

THURSDAY	FRIDAY	SATURDAY	
4	5	**6**	
11	12	**13**	
18	19	**20**	
25	26	**27**	

Feb 1 First Day of Black History Month
Feb 14 Valentine's Day
Feb 15 Presidents' Day (Most regions)

MARCH 2021

SUNDAY	MONDAY	TUESDAY	WEDNESDAY
	1	2	3
7	8	9	10
14	15	16	17
21	22	23	24
28	29	30	31

THURSDAY	FRIDAY	SATURDAY	
4	5	**6**	
11	12	**13**	
18	19	**20**	
25	26	**27**	
			Mar 1 First Day of Women's History Month Mar 17 St. Patrick's Day

APRIL 2021

SUNDAY	MONDAY	TUESDAY	WEDNESDAY
4	5	6	7
11	12	13	14
18	19	20	21
25	26	27	28

THURSDAY	FRIDAY	SATURDAY	
1	2	**3**	
8	9	**10**	
15	16	**17**	
22	23	**24**	
29	30		Apr 4 Easter Sunday Apr 5 Easter Monday Apr 15 Tax Day

MAY 2021

SUNDAY	MONDAY	TUESDAY	WEDNESDAY
2	3	4	5
9	10	11	12
16	17	18	19
23 30	24 31	25	26

THURSDAY	FRIDAY	SATURDAY	
		1	
6	7	**8**	
13	14	**15**	
20	21	**22**	
27	28	**29**	

May 5 Cinco de Mayo
May 9 Mother's Day
May 31 Memorial Day

JUNE 2021

SUNDAY	MONDAY	TUESDAY	WEDNESDAY
		1	2
6	7	8	9
13	14	15	16
20	21	22	23
27	28	29	30

THURSDAY	FRIDAY	SATURDAY	
3	4	**5**	
10	11	**12**	
17	18	**19**	
24	25	**26**	
			Jun 19 Juneteenth Jun 20 Father's Day

JULY 2021

SUNDAY	MONDAY	TUESDAY	WEDNESDAY
4	5	6	7
11	12	13	14
18	19	20	21
25	26	27	28

THURSDAY	FRIDAY	SATURDAY	
1	2	3	
8	9	10	
15	16	17	
22	23	24	
29	30	31	

Jul 4 Independence Day
Jul 5 Independence Day observed

AUGUST 2021

SUNDAY	MONDAY	TUESDAY	WEDNESDAY
1	2	3	4
8	9	10	11
15	16	17	18
22	23	24	25
29	30	31	

THURSDAY	FRIDAY	SATURDAY	
5	6	**7**	
12	13	**14**	
19	20	**21**	
26	27	**28**	

SEPTEMBER 2021

SUNDAY	MONDAY	TUESDAY	WEDNESDAY
			1
5	6	7	8
12	13	14	15
19	20	21	22
26	27	28	29

THURSDAY	FRIDAY	SATURDAY	
2	3	**4**	
9	10	**11**	
16	17	**18**	
23	24	**25**	
30			Sep 6 Labor Day

OCTOBER 2021

SUNDAY	MONDAY	TUESDAY	WEDNESDAY
3	4	5	6
10	11	12	13
17	18	19	20
24 31	25	26	27

THURSDAY	FRIDAY	SATURDAY	
	1	2	
7	8	9	
14	15	16	
21	22	23	
28	29	30	Oct 11 Columbus Day (Most regions) Oct 31 Halloween

NOVEMBER 2021

SUNDAY	MONDAY	TUESDAY	WEDNESDAY
	1	2	3
7	8	9	10
14	15	16	17
21	22	23	24
28	29	30	

THURSDAY	FRIDAY	SATURDAY	
4	5	6	
11	12	13	
18	19	20	
25	26	27	
			Nov 2 Election Day Nov 11 Veterans Day Nov 25 Thanksgiving Day Nov 26 Black Friday

DECEMBER 2021

SUNDAY	MONDAY	TUESDAY	WEDNESDAY
			1
5	6	7	8
12	13	14	15
19	20	21	22
26	27	28	29

THURSDAY	FRIDAY	SATURDAY	
2	3	4	
9	10	11	
16	17	18	
23	24	25	
30	31		

Dec 24 Christmas Day observed
Dec 24 Christmas Eve
Dec 25 Christmas Day
Dec 31 New Year's Day observed
Dec 31 New Year's Eve

WEEK 1
DECEMBER 28, 2020 – JANUARY 3, 2021

WEIGHT :

MONDAY
December 28, 2020

DISTANCE :
TIME :
PACE :
HEART RATE :
CALORIES :

TUESDAY
December 29, 2020

DISTANCE :
TIME :
PACE :
HEART RATE :
CALORIES :

WEDNESDAY
December 30, 2020

DISTANCE :
TIME :
PACE :
HEART RATE :
CALORIES :

THURSDAY
December 31, 2020
New Year's Eve

DISTANCE :
TIME :
PACE :
HEART RATE :
CALORIES :

FRIDAY
January 1, 2021
New Year's Day

DISTANCE :
TIME :
PACE :
HEART RATE :
CALORIES :

SATURDAY
January 2, 2021

DISTANCE :
TIME :
PACE :
HEART RATE :
CALORIES :

SUNDAY
January 3, 2021

DISTANCE :
TIME :
PACE :
HEART RATE :
CALORIES :

TOTAL DISTANCE (FROM LAST WEEK)	
DISTANCE THIS WEEK	
TOTAL DISTANCE	

WEIGHT:

MONDAY
January 4, 2021

DISTANCE:
TIME:
PACE:
HEART RATE:
CALORIES:

TUESDAY
January 5, 2021

DISTANCE:
TIME:
PACE:
HEART RATE:
CALORIES:

WEDNESDAY
January 6, 2021

DISTANCE:
TIME:
PACE:
HEART RATE:
CALORIES:

THURSDAY
January 7, 2021

DISTANCE:
TIME:
PACE:
HEART RATE:
CALORIES:

FRIDAY
January 8, 2021

DISTANCE:
TIME:
PACE:
HEART RATE:
CALORIES:

SATURDAY
January 9, 2021

DISTANCE:
TIME:
PACE:
HEART RATE:
CALORIES:

SUNDAY
January 10, 2021

DISTANCE:
TIME:
PACE:
HEART RATE:
CALORIES:

TOTAL DISTANCE (FROM LAST WEEK)	
DISTANCE THIS WEEK	
TOTAL DISTANCE	

WEEK 3
JANUARY 11, 2021 – JANUARY 17, 2021

WEIGHT :

MONDAY
January 11, 2021

DISTANCE :
TIME :
PACE :
HEART RATE :
CALORIES :

TUESDAY
January 12, 2021

DISTANCE :
TIME :
PACE :
HEART RATE :
CALORIES :

WEDNESDAY
January 13, 2021

DISTANCE :
TIME :
PACE :
HEART RATE :
CALORIES :

THURSDAY
January 14, 2021

DISTANCE :
TIME :
PACE :
HEART RATE :
CALORIES :

FRIDAY
January 15, 2021

DISTANCE :
TIME :
PACE :
HEART RATE :
CALORIES :

SATURDAY
January 16, 2021

DISTANCE :
TIME :
PACE :
HEART RATE :
CALORIES :

SUNDAY
January 17, 2021

DISTANCE :
TIME :
PACE :
HEART RATE :
CALORIES :

TOTAL DISTANCE (FROM LAST WEEK)	
DISTANCE THIS WEEK	
TOTAL DISTANCE	

WEIGHT:

MONDAY
January 18, 2021
Martin Luther King Jr. Day

DISTANCE:
TIME:
PACE:
HEART RATE:
CALORIES:

TUESDAY
January 19, 2021

DISTANCE:
TIME:
PACE:
HEART RATE:
CALORIES:

WEDNESDAY
January 20, 2021

DISTANCE:
TIME:
PACE:
HEART RATE:
CALORIES:

THURSDAY
January 21, 2021

DISTANCE:
TIME:
PACE:
HEART RATE:
CALORIES:

FRIDAY
January 22, 2021

DISTANCE:
TIME:
PACE:
HEART RATE:
CALORIES:

SATURDAY
January 23, 2021

DISTANCE:
TIME:
PACE:
HEART RATE:
CALORIES:

SUNDAY
January 24, 2021

DISTANCE:
TIME:
PACE:
HEART RATE:
CALORIES:

TOTAL DISTANCE (FROM LAST WEEK)	
DISTANCE THIS WEEK	
TOTAL DISTANCE	

WEEK 5
JANUARY 25, 2021 – JANUARY 31, 2021

WEIGHT :

MONDAY
January 25, 2021

DISTANCE :
TIME :
PACE :
HEART RATE :
CALORIES :

TUESDAY
January 26, 2021

DISTANCE :
TIME :
PACE :
HEART RATE :
CALORIES :

WEDNESDAY
January 27, 2021

DISTANCE :
TIME :
PACE :
HEART RATE :
CALORIES :

THURSDAY
January 28, 2021

DISTANCE :
TIME :
PACE :
HEART RATE :
CALORIES :

FRIDAY
January 29, 2021

DISTANCE :
TIME :
PACE :
HEART RATE :
CALORIES :

SATURDAY
January 30, 2021

DISTANCE :
TIME :
PACE :
HEART RATE :
CALORIES :

SUNDAY
January 31, 2021

DISTANCE :
TIME :
PACE :
HEART RATE :
CALORIES :

TOTAL DISTANCE (FROM LAST WEEK)	
DISTANCE THIS WEEK	
TOTAL DISTANCE	

WEIGHT :

MONDAY
February 1, 2021
First Day of Black History Month

DISTANCE :
TIME :
PACE :
HEART RATE :
CALORIES :

TUESDAY
February 2, 2021

DISTANCE :
TIME :
PACE :
HEART RATE :
CALORIES :

WEDNESDAY
February 3, 2021

DISTANCE :
TIME :
PACE :
HEART RATE :
CALORIES :

THURSDAY
February 4, 2021

DISTANCE :
TIME :
PACE :
HEART RATE :
CALORIES :

FRIDAY
February 5, 2021

DISTANCE :
TIME :
PACE :
HEART RATE :
CALORIES :

SATURDAY
February 6, 2021

DISTANCE :
TIME :
PACE :
HEART RATE :
CALORIES :

SUNDAY
February 7, 2021

DISTANCE :
TIME :
PACE :
HEART RATE :
CALORIES :

TOTAL DISTANCE (FROM LAST WEEK)	
DISTANCE THIS WEEK	
TOTAL DISTANCE	

WEEK 7
FEBRUARY 8, 2021 – FEBRUARY 14, 2021

WEIGHT :

MONDAY
February 8, 2021

DISTANCE :
TIME :
PACE :
HEART RATE :
CALORIES :

TUESDAY
February 9, 2021

DISTANCE :
TIME :
PACE :
HEART RATE :
CALORIES :

WEDNESDAY
February 10, 2021

DISTANCE :
TIME :
PACE :
HEART RATE :
CALORIES :

THURSDAY
February 11, 2021

DISTANCE :
TIME :
PACE :
HEART RATE :
CALORIES :

FRIDAY
February 12, 2021

DISTANCE :
TIME :
PACE :
HEART RATE :
CALORIES :

SATURDAY
February 13, 2021

DISTANCE :
TIME :
PACE :
HEART RATE :
CALORIES :

SUNDAY
February 14, 2021
Valentine's Day

DISTANCE :
TIME :
PACE :
HEART RATE :
CALORIES :

TOTAL DISTANCE (FROM LAST WEEK)	
DISTANCE THIS WEEK	
TOTAL DISTANCE	

WEIGHT:

MONDAY
February 15, 2021
Presidents' Day (Most regions)

DISTANCE:
TIME:
PACE:
HEART RATE:
CALORIES:

TUESDAY
February 16, 2021

DISTANCE:
TIME:
PACE:
HEART RATE:
CALORIES:

WEDNESDAY
February 17, 2021

DISTANCE:
TIME:
PACE:
HEART RATE:
CALORIES:

THURSDAY
February 18, 2021

DISTANCE:
TIME:
PACE:
HEART RATE:
CALORIES:

FRIDAY
February 19, 2021

DISTANCE:
TIME:
PACE:
HEART RATE:
CALORIES:

SATURDAY
February 20, 2021

DISTANCE:
TIME:
PACE:
HEART RATE:
CALORIES:

SUNDAY
February 21, 2021

DISTANCE:
TIME:
PACE:
HEART RATE:
CALORIES:

TOTAL DISTANCE (FROM LAST WEEK)	
DISTANCE THIS WEEK	
TOTAL DISTANCE	

WEEK 9
FEBRUARY 22, 2021 – FEBRUARY 28, 2021

WEIGHT :

MONDAY
February 22, 2021

DISTANCE :
TIME :
PACE :
HEART RATE :
CALORIES :

TUESDAY
February 23, 2021

DISTANCE :
TIME :
PACE :
HEART RATE :
CALORIES :

WEDNESDAY
February 24, 2021

DISTANCE :
TIME :
PACE :
HEART RATE :
CALORIES :

THURSDAY
February 25, 2021

DISTANCE :
TIME :
PACE :
HEART RATE :
CALORIES :

FRIDAY
February 26, 2021

DISTANCE :
TIME :
PACE :
HEART RATE :
CALORIES :

SATURDAY
February 27, 2021

DISTANCE :
TIME :
PACE :
HEART RATE :
CALORIES :

SUNDAY
February 28, 2021

DISTANCE :
TIME :
PACE :
HEART RATE :
CALORIES :

TOTAL DISTANCE (FROM LAST WEEK)	
DISTANCE THIS WEEK	
TOTAL DISTANCE	

WEIGHT :

MONDAY
March 1, 2021
First Day of Women's History Month

DISTANCE :
TIME :
PACE :
HEART RATE :
CALORIES :

TUESDAY
March 2, 2021

DISTANCE :
TIME :
PACE :
HEART RATE :
CALORIES :

WEDNESDAY
March 3, 2021

DISTANCE :
TIME :
PACE :
HEART RATE :
CALORIES :

THURSDAY
March 4, 2021

DISTANCE :
TIME :
PACE :
HEART RATE :
CALORIES :

FRIDAY
March 5, 2021

DISTANCE :
TIME :
PACE :
HEART RATE :
CALORIES :

SATURDAY
March 6, 2021

DISTANCE :
TIME :
PACE :
HEART RATE :
CALORIES :

SUNDAY
March 7, 2021

DISTANCE :
TIME :
PACE :
HEART RATE :
CALORIES :

TOTAL DISTANCE (FROM LAST WEEK)	
DISTANCE THIS WEEK	
TOTAL DISTANCE	

WEEK 11
MARCH 8, 2021 – MARCH 14, 2021

WEIGHT :

MONDAY
March 8, 2021

DISTANCE :
TIME :
PACE :
HEART RATE :
CALORIES :

TUESDAY
March 9, 2021

DISTANCE :
TIME :
PACE :
HEART RATE :
CALORIES :

WEDNESDAY
March 10, 2021

DISTANCE :
TIME :
PACE :
HEART RATE :
CALORIES :

THURSDAY
March 11, 2021

DISTANCE :
TIME :
PACE :
HEART RATE :
CALORIES :

FRIDAY
March 12, 2021

DISTANCE :
TIME :
PACE :
HEART RATE :
CALORIES :

SATURDAY
March 13, 2021

DISTANCE :
TIME :
PACE :
HEART RATE :
CALORIES :

SUNDAY
March 14, 2021

DISTANCE :
TIME :
PACE :
HEART RATE :
CALORIES :

TOTAL DISTANCE (FROM LAST WEEK)	
DISTANCE THIS WEEK	
TOTAL DISTANCE	

MONDAY
March 15, 2021

DISTANCE:
TIME:
PACE:
HEART RATE:
CALORIES:

TUESDAY
March 16, 2021

DISTANCE:
TIME:
PACE:
HEART RATE:
CALORIES:

WEDNESDAY
March 17, 2021
St. Patrick's Day

DISTANCE:
TIME:
PACE:
HEART RATE:
CALORIES:

THURSDAY
March 18, 2021

DISTANCE:
TIME:
PACE:
HEART RATE:
CALORIES:

FRIDAY
March 19, 2021

DISTANCE:
TIME:
PACE:
HEART RATE:
CALORIES:

SATURDAY
March 20, 2021

DISTANCE:
TIME:
PACE:
HEART RATE:
CALORIES:

SUNDAY
March 21, 2021

DISTANCE:
TIME:
PACE:
HEART RATE:
CALORIES:

TOTAL DISTANCE (FROM LAST WEEK)	
DISTANCE THIS WEEK	
TOTAL DISTANCE	

WEEK 13
MARCH 22, 2021 – MARCH 28, 2021

WEIGHT :

MONDAY
March 22, 2021

DISTANCE :
TIME :
PACE :
HEART RATE :
CALORIES :

TUESDAY
March 23, 2021

DISTANCE :
TIME :
PACE :
HEART RATE :
CALORIES :

WEDNESDAY
March 24, 2021

DISTANCE :
TIME :
PACE :
HEART RATE :
CALORIES :

THURSDAY
March 25, 2021

DISTANCE :
TIME :
PACE :
HEART RATE :
CALORIES :

FRIDAY
March 26, 2021

DISTANCE :
TIME :
PACE :
HEART RATE :
CALORIES :

SATURDAY
March 27, 2021

DISTANCE :
TIME :
PACE :
HEART RATE :
CALORIES :

SUNDAY
March 28, 2021

DISTANCE :
TIME :
PACE :
HEART RATE :
CALORIES :

TOTAL DISTANCE (FROM LAST WEEK)	
DISTANCE THIS WEEK	
TOTAL DISTANCE	

WEIGHT :

WEEK 14
MARCH 29, 2021 - APRIL 4, 2021

MONDAY
March 29, 2021

DISTANCE :
TIME :
PACE :
HEART RATE :
CALORIES :

TUESDAY
March 30, 2021

DISTANCE :
TIME :
PACE :
HEART RATE :
CALORIES :

WEDNESDAY
March 31, 2021

DISTANCE :
TIME :
PACE :
HEART RATE :
CALORIES :

THURSDAY
April 1, 2021

DISTANCE :
TIME :
PACE :
HEART RATE :
CALORIES :

FRIDAY
April 2, 2021

DISTANCE :
TIME :
PACE :
HEART RATE :
CALORIES :

SATURDAY
April 3, 2021

DISTANCE :
TIME :
PACE :
HEART RATE :
CALORIES :

SUNDAY
April 4, 2021
Easter Sunday

DISTANCE :
TIME :
PACE :
HEART RATE :
CALORIES :

TOTAL DISTANCE (FROM LAST WEEK)	
DISTANCE THIS WEEK	
TOTAL DISTANCE	

WEEK 15
APRIL 5, 2021 – APRIL 11, 2021

WEIGHT :

MONDAY
April 5, 2021
Easter Monday

DISTANCE :
TIME :
PACE :
HEART RATE :
CALORIES :

TUESDAY
April 6, 2021

DISTANCE :
TIME :
PACE :
HEART RATE :
CALORIES :

WEDNESDAY
April 7, 2021

DISTANCE :
TIME :
PACE :
HEART RATE :
CALORIES :

THURSDAY
April 8, 2021

DISTANCE :
TIME :
PACE :
HEART RATE :
CALORIES :

FRIDAY
April 9, 2021

DISTANCE :
TIME :
PACE :
HEART RATE :
CALORIES :

SATURDAY
April 10, 2021

DISTANCE :
TIME :
PACE :
HEART RATE :
CALORIES :

SUNDAY
April 11, 2021

DISTANCE :
TIME :
PACE :
HEART RATE :
CALORIES :

TOTAL DISTANCE (FROM LAST WEEK)	
DISTANCE THIS WEEK	
TOTAL DISTANCE	

WEIGHT:

MONDAY
April 12, 2021

DISTANCE:
TIME:
PACE:
HEART RATE:
CALORIES:

TUESDAY
April 13, 2021

DISTANCE:
TIME:
PACE:
HEART RATE:
CALORIES:

WEDNESDAY
April 14, 2021

DISTANCE:
TIME:
PACE:
HEART RATE:
CALORIES:

THURSDAY
April 15, 2021
Tax Day

DISTANCE:
TIME:
PACE:
HEART RATE:
CALORIES:

FRIDAY
April 16, 2021

DISTANCE:
TIME:
PACE:
HEART RATE:
CALORIES:

SATURDAY
April 17, 2021

DISTANCE:
TIME:
PACE:
HEART RATE:
CALORIES:

SUNDAY
April 18, 2021

DISTANCE:
TIME:
PACE:
HEART RATE:
CALORIES:

TOTAL DISTANCE (FROM LAST WEEK)	
DISTANCE THIS WEEK	
TOTAL DISTANCE	

WEEK 17
APRIL 19, 2021 – APRIL 25, 2021

WEIGHT :

MONDAY
April 19, 2021

DISTANCE :
TIME :
PACE :
HEART RATE :
CALORIES :

TUESDAY
April 20, 2021

DISTANCE :
TIME :
PACE :
HEART RATE :
CALORIES :

WEDNESDAY
April 21, 2021

DISTANCE :
TIME :
PACE :
HEART RATE :
CALORIES :

THURSDAY
April 22, 2021

DISTANCE :
TIME :
PACE :
HEART RATE :
CALORIES :

FRIDAY
April 23, 2021

DISTANCE :
TIME :
PACE :
HEART RATE :
CALORIES :

SATURDAY
April 24, 2021

DISTANCE :
TIME :
PACE :
HEART RATE :
CALORIES :

SUNDAY
April 25, 2021

DISTANCE :
TIME :
PACE :
HEART RATE :
CALORIES :

TOTAL DISTANCE (FROM LAST WEEK)	
DISTANCE THIS WEEK	
TOTAL DISTANCE	

WEIGHT:

MONDAY
April 26, 2021

DISTANCE:
TIME:
PACE:
HEART RATE:
CALORIES:

TUESDAY
April 27, 2021

DISTANCE:
TIME:
PACE:
HEART RATE:
CALORIES:

WEDNESDAY
April 28, 2021

DISTANCE:
TIME:
PACE:
HEART RATE:
CALORIES:

THURSDAY
April 29, 2021

DISTANCE:
TIME:
PACE:
HEART RATE:
CALORIES:

FRIDAY
April 30, 2021

DISTANCE:
TIME:
PACE:
HEART RATE:
CALORIES:

SATURDAY
May 1, 2021

DISTANCE:
TIME:
PACE:
HEART RATE:
CALORIES:

SUNDAY
May 2, 2021

DISTANCE:
TIME:
PACE:
HEART RATE:
CALORIES:

TOTAL DISTANCE (FROM LAST WEEK)	
DISTANCE THIS WEEK	
TOTAL DISTANCE	

WEEK 19
MAY 3, 2021 – MAY 9, 2021

WEIGHT :

MONDAY
May 3, 2021

DISTANCE :
TIME :
PACE :
HEART RATE :
CALORIES :

TUESDAY
May 4, 2021

DISTANCE :
TIME :
PACE :
HEART RATE :
CALORIES :

WEDNESDAY
May 5, 2021
Cinco de Mayo

DISTANCE :
TIME :
PACE :
HEART RATE :
CALORIES :

THURSDAY
May 6, 2021

DISTANCE :
TIME :
PACE :
HEART RATE :
CALORIES :

FRIDAY
May 7, 2021

DISTANCE :
TIME :
PACE :
HEART RATE :
CALORIES :

SATURDAY
May 8, 2021

DISTANCE :
TIME :
PACE :
HEART RATE :
CALORIES :

SUNDAY
May 9, 2021
Mother's Day

DISTANCE :
TIME :
PACE :
HEART RATE :
CALORIES :

TOTAL DISTANCE (FROM LAST WEEK)	
DISTANCE THIS WEEK	
TOTAL DISTANCE	

WEIGHT:

MONDAY
May 10, 2021

DISTANCE:
TIME:
PACE:
HEART RATE:
CALORIES:

TUESDAY
May 11, 2021

DISTANCE:
TIME:
PACE:
HEART RATE:
CALORIES:

WEDNESDAY
May 12, 2021

DISTANCE:
TIME:
PACE:
HEART RATE:
CALORIES:

THURSDAY
May 13, 2021

DISTANCE:
TIME:
PACE:
HEART RATE:
CALORIES:

FRIDAY
May 14, 2021

DISTANCE:
TIME:
PACE:
HEART RATE:
CALORIES:

SATURDAY
May 15, 2021

DISTANCE:
TIME:
PACE:
HEART RATE:
CALORIES:

SUNDAY
May 16, 2021

DISTANCE:
TIME:
PACE:
HEART RATE:
CALORIES:

TOTAL DISTANCE (FROM LAST WEEK)	
DISTANCE THIS WEEK	
TOTAL DISTANCE	

WEEK 21
MAY 17, 2021 – MAY 23, 2021

WEIGHT :

MONDAY
May 17, 2021

DISTANCE :
TIME :
PACE :
HEART RATE :
CALORIES :

TUESDAY
May 18, 2021

DISTANCE :
TIME :
PACE :
HEART RATE :
CALORIES :

WEDNESDAY
May 19, 2021

DISTANCE :
TIME :
PACE :
HEART RATE :
CALORIES :

THURSDAY
May 20, 2021

DISTANCE :
TIME :
PACE :
HEART RATE :
CALORIES :

FRIDAY
May 21, 2021

DISTANCE :
TIME :
PACE :
HEART RATE :
CALORIES :

SATURDAY
May 22, 2021

DISTANCE :
TIME :
PACE :
HEART RATE :
CALORIES :

SUNDAY
May 23, 2021

DISTANCE :
TIME :
PACE :
HEART RATE :
CALORIES :

TOTAL DISTANCE (FROM LAST WEEK)	
DISTANCE THIS WEEK	
TOTAL DISTANCE	

WEIGHT:

MONDAY
May 24, 2021

DISTANCE:
TIME:
PACE:
HEART RATE:
CALORIES:

TUESDAY
May 25, 2021

DISTANCE:
TIME:
PACE:
HEART RATE:
CALORIES:

WEDNESDAY
May 26, 2021

DISTANCE:
TIME:
PACE:
HEART RATE:
CALORIES:

THURSDAY
May 27, 2021

DISTANCE:
TIME:
PACE:
HEART RATE:
CALORIES:

FRIDAY
May 28, 2021

DISTANCE:
TIME:
PACE:
HEART RATE:
CALORIES:

SATURDAY
May 29, 2021

DISTANCE:
TIME:
PACE:
HEART RATE:
CALORIES:

SUNDAY
May 30, 2021

DISTANCE:
TIME:
PACE:
HEART RATE:
CALORIES:

TOTAL DISTANCE (FROM LAST WEEK)	
DISTANCE THIS WEEK	
TOTAL DISTANCE	

WEEK 23
MAY 31, 2021 – JUNE 6, 2021

WEIGHT :

MONDAY
May 31, 2021
Memorial Day

DISTANCE :
TIME :
PACE :
HEART RATE :
CALORIES :

TUESDAY
June 1, 2021

DISTANCE :
TIME :
PACE :
HEART RATE :
CALORIES :

WEDNESDAY
June 2, 2021

DISTANCE :
TIME :
PACE :
HEART RATE :
CALORIES :

THURSDAY
June 3, 2021

DISTANCE :
TIME :
PACE :
HEART RATE :
CALORIES :

FRIDAY
June 4, 2021

DISTANCE :
TIME :
PACE :
HEART RATE :
CALORIES :

SATURDAY
June 5, 2021

DISTANCE :
TIME :
PACE :
HEART RATE :
CALORIES :

SUNDAY
June 6, 2021

DISTANCE :
TIME :
PACE :
HEART RATE :
CALORIES :

TOTAL DISTANCE (FROM LAST WEEK)	
DISTANCE THIS WEEK	
TOTAL DISTANCE	

WEIGHT:

MONDAY
June 7, 2021

DISTANCE:
TIME:
PACE:
HEART RATE:
CALORIES:

TUESDAY
June 8, 2021

DISTANCE:
TIME:
PACE:
HEART RATE:
CALORIES:

WEDNESDAY
June 9, 2021

DISTANCE:
TIME:
PACE:
HEART RATE:
CALORIES:

THURSDAY
June 10, 2021

DISTANCE:
TIME:
PACE:
HEART RATE:
CALORIES:

FRIDAY
June 11, 2021

DISTANCE:
TIME:
PACE:
HEART RATE:
CALORIES:

SATURDAY
June 12, 2021

DISTANCE:
TIME:
PACE:
HEART RATE:
CALORIES:

SUNDAY
June 13, 2021

DISTANCE:
TIME:
PACE:
HEART RATE:
CALORIES:

TOTAL DISTANCE (FROM LAST WEEK)	
DISTANCE THIS WEEK	
TOTAL DISTANCE	

WEEK 25
JUNE 14, 2021 – JUNE 20, 2021

WEIGHT :

MONDAY
June 14, 2021

DISTANCE :
TIME :
PACE :
HEART RATE :
CALORIES :

TUESDAY
June 15, 2021

DISTANCE :
TIME :
PACE :
HEART RATE :
CALORIES :

WEDNESDAY
June 16, 2021

DISTANCE :
TIME :
PACE :
HEART RATE :
CALORIES :

THURSDAY
June 17, 2021

DISTANCE :
TIME :
PACE :
HEART RATE :
CALORIES :

FRIDAY
June 18, 2021

DISTANCE :
TIME :
PACE :
HEART RATE :
CALORIES :

SATURDAY
June 19, 2021
Juneteenth

DISTANCE :
TIME :
PACE :
HEART RATE :
CALORIES :

SUNDAY
June 20, 2021
Father's Day

DISTANCE :
TIME :
PACE :
HEART RATE :
CALORIES :

TOTAL DISTANCE (FROM LAST WEEK)	
DISTANCE THIS WEEK	
TOTAL DISTANCE	

MONDAY
June 21, 2021

DISTANCE:
TIME:
PACE:
HEART RATE:
CALORIES:

TUESDAY
June 22, 2021

DISTANCE:
TIME:
PACE:
HEART RATE:
CALORIES:

WEDNESDAY
June 23, 2021

DISTANCE:
TIME:
PACE:
HEART RATE:
CALORIES:

THURSDAY
June 24, 2021

DISTANCE:
TIME:
PACE:
HEART RATE:
CALORIES:

FRIDAY
June 25, 2021

DISTANCE:
TIME:
PACE:
HEART RATE:
CALORIES:

SATURDAY
June 26, 2021

DISTANCE:
TIME:
PACE:
HEART RATE:
CALORIES:

SUNDAY
June 27, 2021

DISTANCE:
TIME:
PACE:
HEART RATE:
CALORIES:

TOTAL DISTANCE (FROM LAST WEEK)	
DISTANCE THIS WEEK	
TOTAL DISTANCE	

WEEK 27
JUNE 28, 2021 – JULY 4, 2021

WEIGHT :

MONDAY
June 28, 2021

DISTANCE :
TIME :
PACE :
HEART RATE :
CALORIES :

TUESDAY
June 29, 2021

DISTANCE :
TIME :
PACE :
HEART RATE :
CALORIES :

WEDNESDAY
June 30, 2021

DISTANCE :
TIME :
PACE :
HEART RATE :
CALORIES :

THURSDAY
July 1, 2021

DISTANCE :
TIME :
PACE :
HEART RATE :
CALORIES :

FRIDAY
July 2, 2021

DISTANCE :
TIME :
PACE :
HEART RATE :
CALORIES :

SATURDAY
July 3, 2021

DISTANCE :
TIME :
PACE :
HEART RATE :
CALORIES :

SUNDAY
July 4, 2021
Independence Day

DISTANCE :
TIME :
PACE :
HEART RATE :
CALORIES :

TOTAL DISTANCE (FROM LAST WEEK)	
DISTANCE THIS WEEK	
TOTAL DISTANCE	

WEIGHT:

MONDAY
July 5, 2021
Independence Day observed

DISTANCE:
TIME:
PACE:
HEART RATE:
CALORIES:

TUESDAY
July 6, 2021

DISTANCE:
TIME:
PACE:
HEART RATE:
CALORIES:

WEDNESDAY
July 7, 2021

DISTANCE:
TIME:
PACE:
HEART RATE:
CALORIES:

THURSDAY
July 8, 2021

DISTANCE:
TIME:
PACE:
HEART RATE:
CALORIES:

FRIDAY
July 9, 2021

DISTANCE:
TIME:
PACE:
HEART RATE:
CALORIES:

SATURDAY
July 10, 2021

DISTANCE:
TIME:
PACE:
HEART RATE:
CALORIES:

SUNDAY
July 11, 2021

DISTANCE:
TIME:
PACE:
HEART RATE:
CALORIES:

TOTAL DISTANCE (FROM LAST WEEK)	
DISTANCE THIS WEEK	
TOTAL DISTANCE	

WEEK 29
JULY 12, 2021 – JULY 18, 2021

WEIGHT:

MONDAY
July 12, 2021

DISTANCE:
TIME:
PACE:
HEART RATE:
CALORIES:

TUESDAY
July 13, 2021

DISTANCE:
TIME:
PACE:
HEART RATE:
CALORIES:

WEDNESDAY
July 14, 2021

DISTANCE:
TIME:
PACE:
HEART RATE:
CALORIES:

THURSDAY
July 15, 2021

DISTANCE:
TIME:
PACE:
HEART RATE:
CALORIES:

FRIDAY
July 16, 2021

DISTANCE:
TIME:
PACE:
HEART RATE:
CALORIES:

SATURDAY
July 17, 2021

DISTANCE:
TIME:
PACE:
HEART RATE:
CALORIES:

SUNDAY
July 18, 2021

DISTANCE:
TIME:
PACE:
HEART RATE:
CALORIES:

TOTAL DISTANCE (FROM LAST WEEK)	
DISTANCE THIS WEEK	
TOTAL DISTANCE	

WEIGHT :

MONDAY
July 19, 2021

DISTANCE :
TIME :
PACE :
HEART RATE :
CALORIES :

TUESDAY
July 20, 2021

DISTANCE :
TIME :
PACE :
HEART RATE :
CALORIES :

WEDNESDAY
July 21, 2021

DISTANCE :
TIME :
PACE :
HEART RATE :
CALORIES :

THURSDAY
July 22, 2021

DISTANCE :
TIME :
PACE :
HEART RATE :
CALORIES :

FRIDAY
July 23, 2021

DISTANCE :
TIME :
PACE :
HEART RATE :
CALORIES :

SATURDAY
July 24, 2021

DISTANCE :
TIME :
PACE :
HEART RATE :
CALORIES :

SUNDAY
July 25, 2021

DISTANCE :
TIME :
PACE :
HEART RATE :
CALORIES :

TOTAL DISTANCE (FROM LAST WEEK)	
DISTANCE THIS WEEK	
TOTAL DISTANCE	

WEEK 31
JULY 26, 2021 - AUGUST 1, 2021

WEIGHT:

MONDAY
July 26, 2021

DISTANCE:
TIME:
PACE:
HEART RATE:
CALORIES:

TUESDAY
July 27, 2021

DISTANCE:
TIME:
PACE:
HEART RATE:
CALORIES:

WEDNESDAY
July 28, 2021

DISTANCE:
TIME:
PACE:
HEART RATE:
CALORIES:

THURSDAY
July 29, 2021

DISTANCE:
TIME:
PACE:
HEART RATE:
CALORIES:

FRIDAY
July 30, 2021

DISTANCE:
TIME:
PACE:
HEART RATE:
CALORIES:

SATURDAY
July 31, 2021

DISTANCE:
TIME:
PACE:
HEART RATE:
CALORIES:

SUNDAY
August 1, 2021

DISTANCE:
TIME:
PACE:
HEART RATE:
CALORIES:

TOTAL DISTANCE (FROM LAST WEEK)	
DISTANCE THIS WEEK	
TOTAL DISTANCE	

WEIGHT:

MONDAY
August 2, 2021

DISTANCE:
TIME:
PACE:
HEART RATE:
CALORIES:

TUESDAY
August 3, 2021

DISTANCE:
TIME:
PACE:
HEART RATE:
CALORIES:

WEDNESDAY
August 4, 2021

DISTANCE:
TIME:
PACE:
HEART RATE:
CALORIES:

THURSDAY
August 5, 2021

DISTANCE:
TIME:
PACE:
HEART RATE:
CALORIES:

FRIDAY
August 6, 2021

DISTANCE:
TIME:
PACE:
HEART RATE:
CALORIES:

SATURDAY
August 7, 2021

DISTANCE:
TIME:
PACE:
HEART RATE:
CALORIES:

SUNDAY
August 8, 2021

DISTANCE:
TIME:
PACE:
HEART RATE:
CALORIES:

TOTAL DISTANCE (FROM LAST WEEK)	
DISTANCE THIS WEEK	
TOTAL DISTANCE	

WEEK 33
AUGUST 9, 2021 – AUGUST 15, 2021

WEIGHT :

MONDAY
August 9, 2021

DISTANCE :
TIME :
PACE :
HEART RATE :
CALORIES :

TUESDAY
August 10, 2021

DISTANCE :
TIME :
PACE :
HEART RATE :
CALORIES :

WEDNESDAY
August 11, 2021

DISTANCE :
TIME :
PACE :
HEART RATE :
CALORIES :

THURSDAY
August 12, 2021

DISTANCE :
TIME :
PACE :
HEART RATE :
CALORIES :

FRIDAY
August 13, 2021

DISTANCE :
TIME :
PACE :
HEART RATE :
CALORIES :

SATURDAY
August 14, 2021

DISTANCE :
TIME :
PACE :
HEART RATE :
CALORIES :

SUNDAY
August 15, 2021

DISTANCE :
TIME :
PACE :
HEART RATE :
CALORIES :

TOTAL DISTANCE (FROM LAST WEEK)	
DISTANCE THIS WEEK	
TOTAL DISTANCE	

WEIGHT:

MONDAY
August 16, 2021

DISTANCE:
TIME:
PACE:
HEART RATE:
CALORIES:

TUESDAY
August 17, 2021

DISTANCE:
TIME:
PACE:
HEART RATE:
CALORIES:

WEDNESDAY
August 18, 2021

DISTANCE:
TIME:
PACE:
HEART RATE:
CALORIES:

THURSDAY
August 19, 2021

DISTANCE:
TIME:
PACE:
HEART RATE:
CALORIES:

FRIDAY
August 20, 2021

DISTANCE:
TIME:
PACE:
HEART RATE:
CALORIES:

SATURDAY
August 21, 2021

DISTANCE:
TIME:
PACE:
HEART RATE:
CALORIES:

SUNDAY
August 22, 2021

DISTANCE:
TIME:
PACE:
HEART RATE:
CALORIES:

TOTAL DISTANCE (FROM LAST WEEK)	
DISTANCE THIS WEEK	
TOTAL DISTANCE	

WEEK 35
AUGUST 23, 2021 – AUGUST 29, 2021

WEIGHT :

MONDAY
August 23, 2021

DISTANCE :
TIME :
PACE :
HEART RATE :
CALORIES :

TUESDAY
August 24, 2021

DISTANCE :
TIME :
PACE :
HEART RATE :
CALORIES :

WEDNESDAY
August 25, 2021

DISTANCE :
TIME :
PACE :
HEART RATE :
CALORIES :

THURSDAY
August 26, 2021

DISTANCE :
TIME :
PACE :
HEART RATE :
CALORIES :

FRIDAY
August 27, 2021

DISTANCE :
TIME :
PACE :
HEART RATE :
CALORIES :

SATURDAY
August 28, 2021

DISTANCE :
TIME :
PACE :
HEART RATE :
CALORIES :

SUNDAY
August 29, 2021

DISTANCE :
TIME :
PACE :
HEART RATE :
CALORIES :

TOTAL DISTANCE (FROM LAST WEEK)	
DISTANCE THIS WEEK	
TOTAL DISTANCE	

WEIGHT:

MONDAY
August 30, 2021

DISTANCE:
TIME:
PACE:
HEART RATE:
CALORIES:

TUESDAY
August 31, 2021

DISTANCE:
TIME:
PACE:
HEART RATE:
CALORIES:

WEDNESDAY
September 1, 2021

DISTANCE:
TIME:
PACE:
HEART RATE:
CALORIES:

THURSDAY
September 2, 2021

DISTANCE:
TIME:
PACE:
HEART RATE:
CALORIES:

FRIDAY
September 3, 2021

DISTANCE:
TIME:
PACE:
HEART RATE:
CALORIES:

SATURDAY
September 4, 2021

DISTANCE:
TIME:
PACE:
HEART RATE:
CALORIES:

SUNDAY
September 5, 2021

DISTANCE:
TIME:
PACE:
HEART RATE:
CALORIES:

TOTAL DISTANCE (FROM LAST WEEK)	
DISTANCE THIS WEEK	
TOTAL DISTANCE	

WEEK 37
SEPTEMBER 6, 2021 - SEPTEMBER 12, 2021

WEIGHT :

MONDAY
September 6, 2021
Labor Day

DISTANCE :
TIME :
PACE :
HEART RATE :
CALORIES :

TUESDAY
September 7, 2021

DISTANCE :
TIME :
PACE :
HEART RATE :
CALORIES :

WEDNESDAY
September 8, 2021

DISTANCE :
TIME :
PACE :
HEART RATE :
CALORIES :

THURSDAY
September 9, 2021

DISTANCE :
TIME :
PACE :
HEART RATE :
CALORIES :

FRIDAY
September 10, 2021

DISTANCE :
TIME :
PACE :
HEART RATE :
CALORIES :

SATURDAY
September 11, 2021

DISTANCE :
TIME :
PACE :
HEART RATE :
CALORIES :

SUNDAY
September 12, 2021

DISTANCE :
TIME :
PACE :
HEART RATE :
CALORIES :

TOTAL DISTANCE (FROM LAST WEEK)	
DISTANCE THIS WEEK	
TOTAL DISTANCE	

MONDAY
September 13, 2021

DISTANCE :
TIME :
PACE :
HEART RATE :
CALORIES :

TUESDAY
September 14, 2021

DISTANCE :
TIME :
PACE :
HEART RATE :
CALORIES :

WEDNESDAY
September 15, 2021

DISTANCE :
TIME :
PACE :
HEART RATE :
CALORIES :

THURSDAY
September 16, 2021

DISTANCE :
TIME :
PACE :
HEART RATE :
CALORIES :

FRIDAY
September 17, 2021

DISTANCE :
TIME :
PACE :
HEART RATE :
CALORIES :

SATURDAY
September 18, 2021

DISTANCE :
TIME :
PACE :
HEART RATE :
CALORIES :

SUNDAY
September 19, 2021

DISTANCE :
TIME :
PACE :
HEART RATE :
CALORIES :

TOTAL DISTANCE (FROM LAST WEEK)	
DISTANCE THIS WEEK	
TOTAL DISTANCE	

WEEK 39
SEPTEMBER 20, 2021 – SEPTEMBER 26, 2021

WEIGHT :

MONDAY
September 20, 2021

DISTANCE :
TIME :
PACE :
HEART RATE :
CALORIES :

TUESDAY
September 21, 2021

DISTANCE :
TIME :
PACE :
HEART RATE :
CALORIES :

WEDNESDAY
September 22, 2021

DISTANCE :
TIME :
PACE :
HEART RATE :
CALORIES :

THURSDAY
September 23, 2021

DISTANCE :
TIME :
PACE :
HEART RATE :
CALORIES :

FRIDAY
September 24, 2021

DISTANCE :
TIME :
PACE :
HEART RATE :
CALORIES :

SATURDAY
September 25, 2021

DISTANCE :
TIME :
PACE :
HEART RATE :
CALORIES :

SUNDAY
September 26, 2021

DISTANCE :
TIME :
PACE :
HEART RATE :
CALORIES :

TOTAL DISTANCE (FROM LAST WEEK)	
DISTANCE THIS WEEK	
TOTAL DISTANCE	

WEIGHT:

MONDAY
September 27, 2021

DISTANCE:
TIME:
PACE:
HEART RATE:
CALORIES:

TUESDAY
September 28, 2021

DISTANCE:
TIME:
PACE:
HEART RATE:
CALORIES:

WEDNESDAY
September 29, 2021

DISTANCE:
TIME:
PACE:
HEART RATE:
CALORIES:

THURSDAY
September 30, 2021

DISTANCE:
TIME:
PACE:
HEART RATE:
CALORIES:

FRIDAY
October 1, 2021

DISTANCE:
TIME:
PACE:
HEART RATE:
CALORIES:

SATURDAY
October 2, 2021

DISTANCE:
TIME:
PACE:
HEART RATE:
CALORIES:

SUNDAY
October 3, 2021

DISTANCE:
TIME:
PACE:
HEART RATE:
CALORIES:

TOTAL DISTANCE (FROM LAST WEEK)	
DISTANCE THIS WEEK	
TOTAL DISTANCE	

WEEK 41
OCTOBER 4, 2021 – OCTOBER 10, 2021

WEIGHT :

MONDAY
October 4, 2021

DISTANCE :
TIME :
PACE :
HEART RATE :
CALORIES :

TUESDAY
October 5, 2021

DISTANCE :
TIME :
PACE :
HEART RATE :
CALORIES :

WEDNESDAY
October 6, 2021

DISTANCE :
TIME :
PACE :
HEART RATE :
CALORIES :

THURSDAY
October 7, 2021

DISTANCE :
TIME :
PACE :
HEART RATE :
CALORIES :

FRIDAY
October 8, 2021

DISTANCE :
TIME :
PACE :
HEART RATE :
CALORIES :

SATURDAY
October 9, 2021

DISTANCE :
TIME :
PACE :
HEART RATE :
CALORIES :

SUNDAY
October 10, 2021

DISTANCE :
TIME :
PACE :
HEART RATE :
CALORIES :

TOTAL DISTANCE (FROM LAST WEEK)	
DISTANCE THIS WEEK	
TOTAL DISTANCE	

WEIGHT:

MONDAY
October 11, 2021
Columbus Day (Most regions)

DISTANCE:
TIME:
PACE:
HEART RATE:
CALORIES:

TUESDAY
October 12, 2021

DISTANCE:
TIME:
PACE:
HEART RATE:
CALORIES:

WEDNESDAY
October 13, 2021

DISTANCE:
TIME:
PACE:
HEART RATE:
CALORIES:

THURSDAY
October 14, 2021

DISTANCE:
TIME:
PACE:
HEART RATE:
CALORIES:

FRIDAY
October 15, 2021

DISTANCE:
TIME:
PACE:
HEART RATE:
CALORIES:

SATURDAY
October 16, 2021

DISTANCE:
TIME:
PACE:
HEART RATE:
CALORIES:

SUNDAY
October 17, 2021

DISTANCE:
TIME:
PACE:
HEART RATE:
CALORIES:

TOTAL DISTANCE (FROM LAST WEEK)	
DISTANCE THIS WEEK	
TOTAL DISTANCE	

WEEK 43
OCTOBER 18, 2021 – OCTOBER 24, 2021

WEIGHT :

MONDAY
October 18, 2021

DISTANCE :
TIME :
PACE :
HEART RATE :
CALORIES :

TUESDAY
October 19, 2021

DISTANCE :
TIME :
PACE :
HEART RATE :
CALORIES :

WEDNESDAY
October 20, 2021

DISTANCE :
TIME :
PACE :
HEART RATE :
CALORIES :

THURSDAY
October 21, 2021

DISTANCE :
TIME :
PACE :
HEART RATE :
CALORIES :

FRIDAY
October 22, 2021

DISTANCE :
TIME :
PACE :
HEART RATE :
CALORIES :

SATURDAY
October 23, 2021

DISTANCE :
TIME :
PACE :
HEART RATE :
CALORIES :

SUNDAY
October 24, 2021

DISTANCE :
TIME :
PACE :
HEART RATE :
CALORIES :

TOTAL DISTANCE (FROM LAST WEEK)	
DISTANCE THIS WEEK	
TOTAL DISTANCE	

WEIGHT:

MONDAY
October 25, 2021

DISTANCE:
TIME:
PACE:
HEART RATE:
CALORIES:

TUESDAY
October 26, 2021

DISTANCE:
TIME:
PACE:
HEART RATE:
CALORIES:

WEDNESDAY
October 27, 2021

DISTANCE:
TIME:
PACE:
HEART RATE:
CALORIES:

THURSDAY
October 28, 2021

DISTANCE:
TIME:
PACE:
HEART RATE:
CALORIES:

FRIDAY
October 29, 2021

DISTANCE:
TIME:
PACE:
HEART RATE:
CALORIES:

SATURDAY
October 30, 2021

DISTANCE:
TIME:
PACE:
HEART RATE:
CALORIES:

SUNDAY
October 31, 2021
Halloween

DISTANCE:
TIME:
PACE:
HEART RATE:
CALORIES:

TOTAL DISTANCE (FROM LAST WEEK)	
DISTANCE THIS WEEK	
TOTAL DISTANCE	

WEEK 45
NOVEMBER 1, 2021 – NOVEMBER 7, 2021

WEIGHT :

MONDAY
November 1, 2021

DISTANCE :
TIME :
PACE :
HEART RATE :
CALORIES :

TUESDAY
November 2, 2021
Election Day

DISTANCE :
TIME :
PACE :
HEART RATE :
CALORIES :

WEDNESDAY
November 3, 2021

DISTANCE :
TIME :
PACE :
HEART RATE :
CALORIES :

THURSDAY
November 4, 2021

DISTANCE :
TIME :
PACE :
HEART RATE :
CALORIES :

FRIDAY
November 5, 2021

DISTANCE :
TIME :
PACE :
HEART RATE :
CALORIES :

SATURDAY
November 6, 2021

DISTANCE :
TIME :
PACE :
HEART RATE :
CALORIES :

SUNDAY
November 7, 2021

DISTANCE :
TIME :
PACE :
HEART RATE :
CALORIES :

TOTAL DISTANCE (FROM LAST WEEK)	
DISTANCE THIS WEEK	
TOTAL DISTANCE	

MONDAY
November 8, 2021

DISTANCE:
TIME:
PACE:
HEART RATE:
CALORIES:

TUESDAY
November 9, 2021

DISTANCE:
TIME:
PACE:
HEART RATE:
CALORIES:

WEDNESDAY
November 10, 2021

DISTANCE:
TIME:
PACE:
HEART RATE:
CALORIES:

THURSDAY
November 11, 2021
Veterans Day

DISTANCE:
TIME:
PACE:
HEART RATE:
CALORIES:

FRIDAY
November 12, 2021

DISTANCE:
TIME:
PACE:
HEART RATE:
CALORIES:

SATURDAY
November 13, 2021

DISTANCE:
TIME:
PACE:
HEART RATE:
CALORIES:

SUNDAY
November 14, 2021

DISTANCE:
TIME:
PACE:
HEART RATE:
CALORIES:

TOTAL DISTANCE (FROM LAST WEEK)	
DISTANCE THIS WEEK	
TOTAL DISTANCE	

WEEK 47
NOVEMBER 15, 2021 - NOVEMBER 21, 2021

WEIGHT :

MONDAY
November 15, 2021

DISTANCE :
TIME :
PACE :
HEART RATE :
CALORIES :

TUESDAY
November 16, 2021

DISTANCE :
TIME :
PACE :
HEART RATE :
CALORIES :

WEDNESDAY
November 17, 2021

DISTANCE :
TIME :
PACE :
HEART RATE :
CALORIES :

THURSDAY
November 18, 2021

DISTANCE :
TIME :
PACE :
HEART RATE :
CALORIES :

FRIDAY
November 19, 2021

DISTANCE :
TIME :
PACE :
HEART RATE :
CALORIES :

SATURDAY
November 20, 2021

DISTANCE :
TIME :
PACE :
HEART RATE :
CALORIES :

SUNDAY
November 21, 2021

DISTANCE :
TIME :
PACE :
HEART RATE :
CALORIES :

TOTAL DISTANCE (FROM LAST WEEK)	
DISTANCE THIS WEEK	
TOTAL DISTANCE	

MONDAY
November 22, 2021

DISTANCE:
TIME:
PACE:
HEART RATE:
CALORIES:

TUESDAY
November 23, 2021

DISTANCE:
TIME:
PACE:
HEART RATE:
CALORIES:

WEDNESDAY
November 24, 2021

DISTANCE:
TIME:
PACE:
HEART RATE:
CALORIES:

THURSDAY
November 25, 2021
Thanksgiving Day

DISTANCE:
TIME:
PACE:
HEART RATE:
CALORIES:

FRIDAY
November 26, 2021
Black Friday

DISTANCE:
TIME:
PACE:
HEART RATE:
CALORIES:

SATURDAY
November 27, 2021

DISTANCE:
TIME:
PACE:
HEART RATE:
CALORIES:

SUNDAY
November 28, 2021

DISTANCE:
TIME:
PACE:
HEART RATE:
CALORIES:

TOTAL DISTANCE (FROM LAST WEEK)	
DISTANCE THIS WEEK	
TOTAL DISTANCE	

WEEK 49
NOVEMBER 29, 2021 – DECEMBER 5, 2021

WEIGHT:

MONDAY
November 29, 2021

DISTANCE:
TIME:
PACE:
HEART RATE:
CALORIES:

TUESDAY
November 30, 2021

DISTANCE:
TIME:
PACE:
HEART RATE:
CALORIES:

WEDNESDAY
December 1, 2021

DISTANCE:
TIME:
PACE:
HEART RATE:
CALORIES:

THURSDAY
December 2, 2021

DISTANCE:
TIME:
PACE:
HEART RATE:
CALORIES:

FRIDAY
December 3, 2021

DISTANCE:
TIME:
PACE:
HEART RATE:
CALORIES:

SATURDAY
December 4, 2021

DISTANCE:
TIME:
PACE:
HEART RATE:
CALORIES:

SUNDAY
December 5, 2021

DISTANCE:
TIME:
PACE:
HEART RATE:
CALORIES:

TOTAL DISTANCE (FROM LAST WEEK)	
DISTANCE THIS WEEK	
TOTAL DISTANCE	

WEIGHT :

MONDAY
December 6, 2021

DISTANCE :
TIME :
PACE :
HEART RATE :
CALORIES :

TUESDAY
December 7, 2021

DISTANCE :
TIME :
PACE :
HEART RATE :
CALORIES :

WEDNESDAY
December 8, 2021

DISTANCE :
TIME :
PACE :
HEART RATE :
CALORIES :

THURSDAY
December 9, 2021

DISTANCE :
TIME :
PACE :
HEART RATE :
CALORIES :

FRIDAY
December 10, 2021

DISTANCE :
TIME :
PACE :
HEART RATE :
CALORIES :

SATURDAY
December 11, 2021

DISTANCE :
TIME :
PACE :
HEART RATE :
CALORIES :

SUNDAY
December 12, 2021

DISTANCE :
TIME :
PACE :
HEART RATE :
CALORIES :

TOTAL DISTANCE (FROM LAST WEEK)	
DISTANCE THIS WEEK	
TOTAL DISTANCE	

WEEK 51
DECEMBER 13, 2021 – DECEMBER 19, 2021

WEIGHT :

MONDAY
December 13, 2021

DISTANCE :
TIME :
PACE :
HEART RATE :
CALORIES :

TUESDAY
December 14, 2021

DISTANCE :
TIME :
PACE :
HEART RATE :
CALORIES :

WEDNESDAY
December 15, 2021

DISTANCE :
TIME :
PACE :
HEART RATE :
CALORIES :

THURSDAY
December 16, 2021

DISTANCE :
TIME :
PACE :
HEART RATE :
CALORIES :

FRIDAY
December 17, 2021

DISTANCE :
TIME :
PACE :
HEART RATE :
CALORIES :

SATURDAY
December 18, 2021

DISTANCE :
TIME :
PACE :
HEART RATE :
CALORIES :

SUNDAY
December 19, 2021

DISTANCE :
TIME :
PACE :
HEART RATE :
CALORIES :

TOTAL DISTANCE (FROM LAST WEEK)	
DISTANCE THIS WEEK	
TOTAL DISTANCE	

WEIGHT:

MONDAY
December 20, 2021

DISTANCE:
TIME:
PACE:
HEART RATE:
CALORIES:

TUESDAY
December 21, 2021

DISTANCE:
TIME:
PACE:
HEART RATE:
CALORIES:

WEDNESDAY
December 22, 2021

DISTANCE:
TIME:
PACE:
HEART RATE:
CALORIES:

THURSDAY
December 23, 2021

DISTANCE:
TIME:
PACE:
HEART RATE:
CALORIES:

FRIDAY
December 24, 2021
Christmas Day observed / Christmas Eve

DISTANCE:
TIME:
PACE:
HEART RATE:
CALORIES:

SATURDAY
December 25, 2021
Christmas Day

DISTANCE:
TIME:
PACE:
HEART RATE:
CALORIES:

SUNDAY
December 26, 2021

DISTANCE:
TIME:
PACE:
HEART RATE:
CALORIES:

TOTAL DISTANCE (FROM LAST WEEK)	
DISTANCE THIS WEEK	
TOTAL DISTANCE	

WEEK 53
DECEMBER 27, 2021 – JANUARY 2, 2022

WEIGHT:

MONDAY
December 27, 2021

DISTANCE:
TIME:
PACE:
HEART RATE:
CALORIES:

TUESDAY
December 28, 2021

DISTANCE:
TIME:
PACE:
HEART RATE:
CALORIES:

WEDNESDAY
December 29, 2021

DISTANCE:
TIME:
PACE:
HEART RATE:
CALORIES:

THURSDAY
December 30, 2021

DISTANCE:
TIME:
PACE:
HEART RATE:
CALORIES:

FRIDAY
December 31, 2021
New Year's Day observed / New Year's Eve

DISTANCE:
TIME:
PACE:
HEART RATE:
CALORIES:

SATURDAY
January 1, 2022
New Year's Day

DISTANCE:
TIME:
PACE:
HEART RATE:
CALORIES:

SUNDAY
January 2, 2022

DISTANCE:
TIME:
PACE:
HEART RATE:
CALORIES:

TOTAL DISTANCE (FROM LAST WEEK)	
DISTANCE THIS WEEK	
TOTAL DISTANCE	

Made in the USA
Coppell, TX
02 December 2020

42745853R10066